UNDERSTANDING

GREEEN TEA EXTRACT

AND BENEFITS

A Guide To Boosting Metabolism, Enhancing Cognitive Function, Weight Management, And Achieving Optimal Wellness

DR. LACEY MICHELLE

Copyright © Lacey Michelle 2023

Disclaimer:

The information provided in this book is for general informational purposes only and is not intended as medical advice.

Readers are encouraged to consult with a qualified healthcare professional for any health concerns or questions.

Contents

About The Book

Green tea extract's future as a dietary supplement

Forecasts and Conjectures

Consequences for the Wellness and Health Sector

Suggestions for Further Research

Wrap-Up

Set out on an adventure where research, custom, and useful advice come together to highlight the enormous potential of green tea extract as a pillar in your quest for a happier, better life.

CHAPTER ONE

History And Origin

The history of green tea, which is made from the leaves of the Camellia sinensis plant, is extensive and goes back thousands of years. Its history dates back to ancient China when it was utilized as a medicine and drank as a beverage.

Around 2737 BCE, the fabled Chinese Emperor Shen Nong is frequently credited with discovering tea, notably green tea. The first cup of tea is said to have been made when a tea leaf dropped into a pot of boiling water that he was preparing.

Green tea growing and drinking become firmly embedded in Chinese society over time.

Green tea gained popularity in China during the Tang Dynasty (618–907 CE). Green tea's standing was further enhanced by the "Classic of Tea" (Cha Jing), a book on tea culture and preparation techniques written by the well-known Chinese poet Lu Yu. The development of tea production and processing methods throughout this period laid the foundation for modern green tea.

Eventually, green tea left China and traveled abroad. It arrived in Japan, where it was assimilated into the national identity and customs of the country.

Green tea was first brought to Japan by Buddhist monks, and the preparation and drinking of matcha, or powdered green tea, became the focal point of the Japanese tea ceremony (chanoyu).

The popularity of green tea kept rising in the centuries that followed. It traveled to other Asian countries including Korea and Vietnam. In the early modern era, green tea was brought to the West by European explorers and traders, and it quickly gained popularity. Green tea became more widely known throughout the world as its potential health advantages were realized, and its antioxidant qualities and prospective medical applications were acknowledged.

Green tea is now grown and consumed extensively worldwide. It comes in a variety of forms, from handy tea bags and extracts to loose-leaf teas. The persistent appeal and cultural significance of green tea, together with its path from Chinese mythology to a globally recognized beverage and supplement with possible health advantages, are all demonstrated by its history.

The Science of Extracting Green Tea

Recent years have seen a considerable increase in interest in green tea extract because of its rich mix of bioactive components and potential health benefits. The science of antioxidants, specifically catechins and more precisely epigallocatechin gallate (EGCG), is fundamental to its medicinal benefits.

Green tea extract is a potent and adaptable dietary supplement with many uses in enhancing health and well-being because of these polyphenolic components.

Oxidant Characteristics

Strong antioxidant qualities are the reason for the popularity of green tea extract. Antioxidants are substances that work to mitigate the negative consequences of oxidative stress, which is the process by which the body produces dangerous free radicals.

Unstable chemicals called free radicals can harm DNA, proteins, and cells, which accelerates aging and several chronic illnesses. Numerous antioxidants found in green tea extract work well to scavenge free radicals and lower the chance of cellular damage.

Within the class of polyphenolic chemicals known as catechins, the main antioxidants are found in green tea extract.

Catechins: Their Advantages

Green tea extract contains a class of polyphenols called catechins, among which epicatechin, epicatechin gallate, epigallocatechin, and epigallocatechin gallate

(EGCG) are the most prevalent and thoroughly researched. Strong antioxidants, these catechins provide numerous health advantages.

Their capacity to lower the chance of chronic illnesses, such as cardiovascular conditions and some forms of cancer, is one of their most noteworthy advantages.

Because they lower blood pressure, increase endothelial function, and lower LDL cholesterol levels, catechins have been associated with improved cardiovascular health.

Green tea extract is an important part of weight loss and diabetes management programs because it also shows promise in supporting glucose control and weight management.

CHAPTER TWO

Epigallocatechin Gallate or EGCG

Epigallocatechin gallate (EGCG) is the most bioactive and researched component of the catechins.

Because of its remarkable anti-inflammatory and antioxidant qualities, EGCG has come to be recognized as having medicinal promise.

According to research, EGCG may shield brain tissue from harm, thereby lowering the chance of developing neurodegenerative illnesses like Parkinson's and Alzheimer's.

Furthermore, EGCG has been linked to enhanced metabolism, which makes it a topic of interest for people trying to control their weight and avoid obesity.

Given that EGCG can stop the proliferation of cancer cells and encourage apoptosis, or planned cell death, in malignant tissues, its function in cancer prevention is very significant.

Polyphones And Well-Being

Green tea and other plant-based meals and drinks are rich in polyphenols, a broad class of naturally occurring chemicals. These substances are well known for their capacity to improve health and offer protection from a range of illnesses.

Polyphenols are prevalent in green tea extract and are primarily responsible for its health benefits.

Green tea polyphenols have anti-inflammatory, antibacterial, and cardiovascular-protective qualities in addition to particular catechins like EGCG.

By lowering the risk of chronic illnesses, boosting immunity, and enhancing general metabolic health, they improve people's general well-being.

The strong antioxidant qualities of green tea extract, which are mainly fueled by catechins like EGCG, are the scientific basis for its effectiveness.

Numerous health benefits have been established by these bioactive chemicals, including prospective applications in weight control, cancer prevention, and cardiovascular health, in addition to their antioxidant and anti-inflammatory properties. Packed in polyphenols, green tea extract is a powerful example of how nature has gifted human health.

It may also be used as a beneficial dietary supplement for people who want to improve their overall health and lower their chance of developing chronic illnesses.

Supplements containing green tea extract are made from Camellia sinensis leaves, and because of their high concentration of bioactive chemicals, they provide a wide range of potential health advantages.

These supplements are available in a variety of forms, each with special qualities and attributes of its own. We'll examine some of the most well-liked varieties of green tea extract pills below.

Matcha is a Japanese-style powdered green tea that has been finely ground. It has a distinctive flavor and a vivid green hue. Because the tea leaves used to make matcha are cultivated in shadow, their chlorophyll level and amino acid composition are enhanced.

This variety of green tea extract is well-known for having a high concentration of antioxidants, particularly catechins, which makes it an effective source of substances that are good for you.

In addition to being a common ingredient in traditional Japanese tea ceremonies, matcha can be added to a variety of culinary preparations, including lattes, smoothies, and desserts.

Sencha is the most widely eaten variety of green tea both in Japan and around the world.

Tea leaves cultivated in direct sunlight are used to make it. Sencha, in contrast to matcha, is dried and rolled into needle-like shapes rather than being ground into a powder. Sencha contains a high concentration of catechins, specifically epigallocatechin gallate (EGCG), which has been linked to several health advantages, such as its antioxidant and possibly anti-cancer capabilities. Sencha usually has a grassy, slightly astringent flavor characteristic.

Premium Japanese green tea, gyokuro, is prized for its vivid green color and sweet, umami taste. It is grown in shadow, just like matcha, but the leaves aren't powdered. The chlorophyll level rises during the shading process, giving the product a distinct flavor profile.

Gyokuro is a popular tea among people who value the nuances of green tea because of its delicate and sophisticated flavor. It is linked to possible health advantages and, like other green teas, has a high catechin content.

Japanese green tea genmaicha, sometimes called "popcorn tea," is made by mixing roasted brown rice with green tea leaves. This unusual mix produces a mildly roasted scent along with a nutty flavor.

Because it tastes less harsh than other green teas and because rice adds a unique flavor to the blend, genmaicha is frequently regarded as a friendly and daily option.

Even though its catechin level could be a little lower than that of other green teas, many who enjoy its flavor and scent continue to choose it.

A type of green tea called decaffeinated green tea extract has had the caffeine concentration lowered by this method. Those who are sensitive to caffeine or who want the possible health advantages of green tea without the stimulating effects can use this sort of extract.

While there are differences in decaffeination techniques, the basic goal is to eliminate the majority of the caffeine while leaving behind the health benefits of the tea, such as catechins.

It's important to remember that decaffeinated green tea extract is still a good choice for people who would rather avoid caffeine because it still has antioxidant qualities and other health benefits.

There is a wide variety of tastes, qualities, and possible health advantages offered by the different kinds of green tea extract supplements. There is a green tea variety to fit your tastes and unique health requirements, whether you prefer the intense, rich flavor of matcha, the grassy undertones of sencha, the umami sweetness of gyokuro, the nutty scent of genmaicha, or the caffeine-free alternative of decaffeinated green tea extract.

The distinct attributes that every variety of green tea extract offers to the table add to the general appeal of green tea as a beverage that promotes health.

A well-liked dietary supplement, green tea extract has drawn a lot of interest due to its possible health advantages. The Camellia sinensis plant yields green tea, which is prized for having a high concentration of bioactive substances, especially catechins, which give it potent antioxidant properties. These substances are thought to support numerous health benefits, such as improved metabolism, heart health, brain function, skin and beauty, and weight control.

Weight control is among the most well-known health advantages of green tea extract. Epigallocatechin gallate (EGCG), one type of catechin, can raise metabolism and speed up the body's fat-burning process. Additionally, green tea extract may help suppress appetite, which would make it simpler for people to limit their calorie consumption. For people who want to lose weight and keep it off, these effects may be extremely helpful.

Regarding heart health, green tea extract has demonstrated encouraging possibilities. Regular ingestion of green tea has been associated with a reduction in cardiovascular disease risk variables, including blood pressure, LDL cholesterol, and blood vessel function. The extract's antioxidant qualities help guard against LDL cholesterol oxidation, a major cause of atherosclerosis, a disorder in which fatty deposits build up in the artery walls and cause the walls to harden.

Another area where green tea extract may be beneficial is in the field of brain health. Its bioactive components, especially EGCG, are thought to have neuroprotective qualities that help protect brain cells from oxidative stress-related damage. This defense might help lower the chance of developing neurodegenerative illnesses like Parkinson's and Alzheimer's.

Moreover, increased alertness and better cognitive performance have been linked to green tea extract.

One highly valued advantage of green tea extract is its capacity to increase metabolism. It can help with weight loss and maintaining a healthy body composition by increasing the rate at which the body burns calories. Additionally, it can raise energy expenditure, which facilitates physical activity and amplifies the benefits of exercise for people trying to get fitter and feel better overall.

Green tea extract has several benefits for people who are interested in skin and cosmetic benefits.

Because of its strong antioxidant content, it helps shield the skin from free radical damage, which can create wrinkles fine lines, and other signs of premature aging. Green tea extract has anti-inflammatory qualities that can help reduce redness and irritation of the skin, which makes it a useful component in skincare products.

According to some research, topically using green tea extract may even help lower the chance of developing skin cancer and shield against the damaging effects of UV radiation.

One adaptable supplement with several possible health advantages is green tea extract.

The bioactive components in green tea extract have drawn interest in several health and wellness domains, including weight control, heart health, cognitive function, metabolism enhancement, and benefits for skin and beauty. Individual reactions to the supplement may differ, so before adding it to your daily routine, especially if you have underlying medical conditions or are taking medication, it's best to speak with a healthcare provider.

Antioxidant Properties Of Green Tea Extract

Green tea extract is becoming more well-known for its strong antioxidant qualities. Compounds called antioxidants are essential for shielding the body from the harmful effects of free radicals.

Free radicals are extremely reactive chemicals that can cause oxidative stress, a process linked to aging and several diseases. To fight oxidative stress, green tea, especially its active polyphenols, provides a healthy and efficient source of antioxidants.

Adverse Reactions with Free Radicals

Unpaired electrons create dangerous molecules known as free radicals, which are naturally occurring byproducts of the body's many metabolic activities as well as environmental triggers including pollution, UV radiation exposure, and poor diets.

Oxidative stress can result when the body's supply of antioxidants cannot keep up with the free radicals' numbers.

Numerous health problems, such as cancer, heart disease, and neurological disorders are linked to oxidative stress. Rich in substances like epicatechins, flavonoids, and catechins, green tea extract scavenges these free radicals, lessening their damaging effects and shielding cells from injury.

CHAPTER THREE

Green Tea Extract And Defense Of Cells

Increasing the body's resistance to oxidative stress is one of the main ways that green tea extract delivers its antioxidant benefits.

It supports the delicate equilibrium that exists between antioxidants and free radicals. Green tea's active ingredients can neutralize free radicals and stop them from damaging cells.

Additionally, green tea extract can stimulate several cellular defense mechanisms, including raising the synthesis of antioxidant enzymes like catalase and superoxide dismutase.

The maintenance of cell integrity and health is facilitated by this improved cellular defense, which is essential for general health.

Reverse Aging Effects

The processes of oxidative stress and cellular damage are intimately related to the idea of anti-aging.

Our bodies start to age on the inside as well as the outside as damage to our cells accumulates over time.

Because green tea extract contains antioxidants, it can slow down the aging process by protecting our tissues and cells.

In addition to protecting against age-related illnesses, it may also improve the appearance and health of the skin.

Furthermore, the prevention of fine lines and wrinkles in the skin has been linked to green tea extract.

Since green tea extract can increase skin suppleness and lessen UV-induced skin damage, it is sometimes included in skincare products.

 Green tea's polyphenols can support the maintenance of collagen levels, which are necessary for skin to look youthful.

In this sense, the anti-aging benefits of green tea extract extend beyond internal well-being to include preserving a more youthful and lively outside appearance.

The antioxidant properties of green tea extract play a critical role in preventing oxidative stress, shielding cells, and promoting anti-aging benefits.

Its active ingredients are crucial for preserving cellular health and lessening the harmful effects of free radicals.

Green tea extract, whether ingested as a drink or used in cosmetic products, is still being recognized for its potential to support general health and well-being and maintain a youthful, bright appearance.

CHAPTER FOUR

Green Tea Extract And Preventing Cancer

Because of its possible health benefits, green tea extract is a naturally occurring chemical that is made from the leaves of the Camellia sinensis plant and is frequently drunk as a beverage.

The possibility that green tea extract can prevent cancer is among its most intriguing features. Several investigations have examined the connection between green tea extract and its potential to lower cancer risk.

Investigations And Reports

A significant amount of scientific literature has been devoted to examining the possible cancer-preventive effects of green tea extract. Numerous cancer types have been the subject of studies, including gastrointestinal, lung, prostate, and breast cancers.

There is epidemiological evidence that people who consume a lot of green tea—like those in parts of Asia—have lower cancer incidence rates.

These findings encouraged further thorough research to clarify the underlying mechanisms behind this behavior.

A significant finding of this study is the presence of polyphenolic chemicals, specifically catechins, in green tea. The strong catechin epigallocatechin gallate (EGCG) has attracted a lot of interest because of its possible anticancer effects. EGCG has been shown in numerous studies to prevent the growth of cancer cells, cause apoptosis, or programmed cell death, and prevent angiogenesis—the process of forming new blood vessels to support tumors—from occurring.

Systems Of Action

There are several different ways that green tea extract may prevent cancer. First of all, it has potent antioxidant qualities. Green tea's bioactive ingredients, especially catechins, work as free radical scavengers to scavenge dangerous reactive oxygen species (ROS), which can damage and alter cells.

Green tea extract may help prevent cancer from starting by lowering oxidative stress and DNA damage.

Moreover, it has been shown that green tea extract can modify several signaling pathways that are essential to the development of cancer.

It can prevent the activation of particular transcription factors and enzymes that support the development and viability of cancer cells.

Furthermore, it has been shown that the catechins in green tea inhibit the expression of genes linked to inflammation and cell growth, which may help prevent cancer.

Preventing Oxidative Stress

One of the main causes of cancer development is oxidative damage. Cellular DNA damage and mutations can result from an imbalance between antioxidants and free radicals.

This equilibrium is preserved in part by the abundant antioxidant content of green tea extract. Green tea catechins can stop the accumulation of DNA mutations that might otherwise cause cancer cells to grow out of control by lowering oxidative stress.

Furthermore, green tea extract's anti-inflammatory qualities are significant for preventing cancer. Because chronic inflammation can foster an environment that is conducive to tumor growth, it has been related to the development of cancer. The inflammatory response in cells and tissues can be reduced by green tea catechins, which can suppress pro-inflammatory chemicals and signaling pathways.

Although there is hope for green tea extract's role in cancer prevention, further research is necessary before firm guidelines for its application in clinical settings can be established. Green tea extract ought to be viewed as a component of a more comprehensive cancer prevention plan that also consists of a good diet, frequent exercise, and other lifestyle changes. However, the evidence that is currently available regarding the mechanisms of action—which is backed up by a large number of research studies—underlines the possible advantages of green tea extract in lowering the risk of cancer, which makes it an intriguing topic for oncology research.

CHAPTER FIVE

Green Tea Extract And Controlling Weight

A well-known dietary supplement that has grown in popularity is green tea extract, which may help with weight management.

The leaves of the Camellia sinensis plant, which have been utilized for millennia in traditional medicine because of their numerous health advantages, are the source of this natural product.

The link between green tea extract and weight control is supported by several important processes, including hunger suppression, fat oxidation, thermogenesis, and effects on metabolic rate.

Oxidation Of Fat

The enhancement of fat oxidation is one of the main ways that green tea extract helps with weight management.

Green tea is rich in a class of bioactive substances called catechins, the most prevalent and powerful of which is epigallocatechin gallate (EGCG). It has been demonstrated that EGCG speeds up the body's oxidation of fat for energy, encouraging the body to break down fat reserves. This procedure makes it possible to use body fat as an energy source more effectively, which may prevent fat from accumulating and support weight loss attempts.

Heat-Producing

It is also known that green tea extract encourages thermogenesis, the body's process of producing heat. Thermogenesis has a role in calorie burning and subsequent weight loss.

It has been demonstrated that green tea catechins like EGCG promote thermogenesis, which may raise metabolic rate.

Because of this increased metabolism, people may be able to burn more calories even while they are at rest, which would facilitate effective weight management.

Suppression Of Appetite

The ability of green tea extract to decrease hunger is another way that it may help with weight management.

According to certain research, the chemicals in green tea, such as EGCG, may have an impact on the hormones and neurotransmitters that control hunger. Green tea extract may aid in weight loss efforts by encouraging feelings of fullness, which may lead to people consuming fewer calories throughout the day. Those attempting to regulate their calorie intake and weight may find this appetite suppression very helpful.

Loss Of Weight And Metabolic Rate

The pace at which the body burns calories for energy is called the metabolic rate, and green tea extract has the power to affect it. As was already noted, green tea catechins have a thermogenic impact that can raise metabolic rate and enhance calorie burn.

A greater metabolic rate makes it easier to use fat that has been stored as energy and helps maintain a healthy body weight, over time, this may aid in weight loss. Incorporating green tea extract into a weight management plan can be a helpful and natural way to support weight loss goals and metabolic rate, even though the effect might not be dramatic.

The possible involvement of green tea extract in weight management through different pathways has attracted interest.

It increases thermogenesis, inhibits hunger, accelerates fat oxidation, and modifies metabolic rate. Although it's important to keep in mind that green tea extract is not a miracle weight loss aid and should instead be used in concert with a healthy diet and frequent exercise, taking it as a dietary supplement can provide people with a safe and natural way to help them achieve their weight management goals.

CHAPTER SIX

Green Tea Extract For Mental Well-Being

The potential benefits of green tea extract for cognitive health have drawn a lot of attention in recent years. Green tea extract is associated with improved mood, neuroprotection against Alzheimer's disease, memory and learning, and mood enhancement.

Memory And Learning:

Improving memory and learning skills is one of the main areas of study in how green tea extract affects cognitive health. The potential of green tea's active ingredients, like the amino acid L-theanine and catechins, to improve cognitive function has been researched. These substances might aid in memory consolidation, which would help with information retention and speed up the learning process.

 Furthermore, green tea extract's caffeine level might improve focus and alertness, which may help with memory and learning skills.

Neuroprotection:

Strong antioxidants found in green tea extract, especially epigallocatechin gallate (EGCG), have been shown to have neuroprotective effects.

These antioxidants support the fight against oxidative stress and inflammation in the brain, two major conditions linked to cognitive loss. Green tea extract may increase cognitive function and improve the general health of brain cells by protecting them from damage brought on by free radicals and other dangerous chemicals.

Alzheimer's Disease:

The buildup of tau tangles and beta-amyloid plaques in the brain causes cognitive impairment. Alzheimer's disease is a neurodegenerative disorder.

The possible significance of green tea extract in managing and preventing Alzheimer's disease has been studied. According to certain research, green tea's bioactive components may be able to stop beta-amyloid plaques from forming and lessen their toxicity.

These results suggest that green tea extract may be useful in reducing the risk of Alzheimer's disease, but further research is required.

Enhancement of Mood: Emotional stability and mood play important roles in cognitive health, which extends beyond memory and learning.

Because green tea extract interacts with the central nervous system, it has been associated with improved mood. Green tea contains the amino acid L-theanine, which is well-known for its relaxing and mood-stabilizing properties.

It can boost the synthesis of neurotransmitters like as serotonin and dopamine, which encourage relaxation and enhance mental health in general. Green tea extract's caffeine and L-theanine combination produces a balanced alertness without the jitters, which enhances mood even more.

Green tea extract has the potential to improve cognitive health in several ways. Its importance in maintaining and enhancing cognitive function is highlighted by its capacity to improve memory and learning, offer neuroprotection, and maybe lower the risk of Alzheimer's disease. Green tea extract is a desirable dietary supplement for people who want to preserve and improve their cognitive capacities because it also has mood-enhancing qualities that may support general cognitive well-being.

Although there is still more research to be done, the results of this study indicate that adding green tea extract to a balanced diet could be a useful tactic for enhancing cognitive health.

CHAPTER SEVEN

Green Tea Extract For Beautification And Skin

The potential benefits of green tea extract in boosting skin health and appearance have led to a notable increase in popularity in recent years.

Rich in antioxidants and bioactive components, this natural supplement can improve the condition of your skin in several ways, such as preventing aging indications on your skin, treating acne and other blemishes, and even promoting healthy hair. Green tea extract has other uses outside of oral supplements. It can be mixed with DIY beauty treatments to offer a natural and comprehensive skincare solution.

Strong antioxidants known as catechins, including epigallocatechin gallate (EGCG), are found in green tea extract and may help shield the skin from the damaging effects of free radicals. Unstable chemicals called free radicals have the potential to harm skin cells and hasten the aging process.

Green tea extract can help minimize the appearance of fine lines, wrinkles, and age spots by reducing oxidative stress on the skin by neutralizing these free radicals. Taking green tea extract supplements regularly could help you seem younger and more attractive.

Moreover, the anti-inflammatory qualities of green tea extract might help calm irritated skin and possibly reduce symptoms like redness and puffiness. Because collagen production is necessary to maintain tight and supple skin, it may also help to preserve skin elasticity. Green tea extract can therefore be a beneficial addition to a skincare regimen meant to counteract the signs of aging.

Blotches And Pimples

People of all ages can suffer from acne, and green tea extract may be a natural cure for those who suffer from this skin ailment. The antibacterial qualities of green tea extract can help attack acne-causing germs and reduce the frequency and severity of outbreaks.

Furthermore, green tea extract's anti-inflammatory properties might lessen the redness and swelling brought on by acne.

Furthermore, the polyphenols in green tea extract can control the production of sebum, the skin's natural oil, which can exacerbate acne. Green tea extract helps prevent clogged pores and reduce the appearance of blackheads and whiteheads by regulating sebum production. Green tea extract is a powerful weapon in the fight against acne and pimples; adding supplements to your skincare regimen may promote healthier, smoother skin.

Hair Wellness

Green tea extract has many benefits for skin health, but it can also have several positive effects on hair health. Green tea extract has antioxidants that can help shield hair follicles from damage brought on by free radicals, thereby encouraging the growth of healthy hair. Furthermore, green tea extract includes chemicals that block the hormone dihydrotestosterone (DHT), which is associated with hair loss and thinning. By suppressing DHT, green tea extract may help maintain thicker and fuller hair.

Additionally, green tea extract might improve the overall condition of the scalp. Its anti-inflammatory qualities can reduce flakiness, dryness, and irritation, improving the conditions for hair development. To hydrate your hair and keep it vibrant, think about taking green tea extract supplements or utilizing green tea-based hair products.

Homemade Green Tea Cosmetic Procedures

Green tea extract can be applied topically to improve your beauty regimen in addition to being taken orally. Because green tea is naturally skin-friendly, many people decide to make their own green tea beauty treatments.

A popular do-it-yourself project is a green tea face mask. Green tea extract or brewed green tea can be combined with other natural ingredients like honey, yogurt, or aloe vera gel to form this mask. By using this mask, you may hydrate your skin, lessen inflammation, and enhance its texture.

Making a green tea toner is another option to include green tea in your beauty routine. Green tea extract, water, and a few drops of essential oil can be combined to make a calming and revitalizing toner that balances the pH of the skin and reduces the visibility of pores.

To sum up, green tea extract provides a comprehensive strategy for enhancing skin and beauty. For people looking for a natural solution to improve their looks, this supplement is highly adaptable because of its substantial antioxidant content, anti-inflammatory qualities, and potential advantages for hair health.

Green tea extract can bring significant benefits to your skincare routine, whether it is taken orally or employed in homemade beauty treatments.

CHAPTER EIGHT

How To Pick The Best Extract For Green Tea

With so many options on the market, selecting the best green tea extract supplement can be challenging.

Because it contains a high concentration of bioactive chemicals called catechins, especially epigallocatechin gallate (EGCG), green tea extract is well known for its potential health advantages. But to fully utilize these advantages, it's critical to take into account several variables while choosing a green tea extract supplement.

Qualitative Factors

The selection of the appropriate supplement heavily depends on the quality of the green tea extract. Choose items that are guaranteed to have a certain amount of catechins; those with a higher EGCG concentration are generally preferable. Seek supplements manufactured from premium tea leaves, preferably from respectable places like China, Taiwan, or Japan, which are renowned for their excellent methods of growing tea.

To guarantee that the product satisfies quality standards, independent testing for potency and purity is also essential.

Additionally, take into account if the product is devoid of additives and pollutants. Preservatives, colorants, and artificial fillers ought to be avoided. A product that is cleaner and more natural may be indicated by its organic and non-GMO certifications. Furthermore, monitoring the extraction techniques and storage conditions during the manufacturing process can assist in guaranteeing that the advantageous chemicals in the extract are preserved.

The Administration And Dosage

To reap the potential health benefits of green tea extract while averting its side effects, the right dosage and method of administration must be established.

The suggested dosage may change based on the particular product and the intended result. EGCG is often recommended for people looking to reduce weight and benefit from antioxidants at a dose of 250–500 mg per day. Higher doses, however, can be necessary for therapeutic purposes or particular medical conditions; in such cases, they should be given under a doctor's supervision.

Another important consideration is the time of eating. Supplements containing green tea extract are usually taken with meals to enhance absorption and lower the possibility of upset stomach. However, it's crucial to follow the product's suggested directions and not exceed the given daily dosage, since excessive use might lead to unwanted consequences.

Possible Adverse Reactions

When used as prescribed, green tea extract is usually seen to be safe for most people, but it's vital to be aware of any possible negative effects. Green tea extract contains caffeine, which some people may find too strong. Nervousness, jitters, and sleep difficulties are possible side effects. To avoid affecting your sleep habits, it's best to use decaffeinated versions or time when you take supplements.

Higher dosages of green tea extract have occasionally been linked to digestive problems like upset stomachs and diarrhea. These negative effects could be mitigated by changing products or adjusting the dosage.

Before taking green tea extract supplements, people with specific medical conditions, such as liver illness, or those who are sensitive to catechins should speak with a healthcare provider because taking too much of it can be hazardous to the liver.

Quality, dose, and potential adverse effects must all be carefully considered when selecting a green tea extract product. Through quality prioritization, adherence to appropriate dosages, and awareness of potential side effects, people can optimize the health advantages of these supplements while reducing the dangers.

Before beginning a new supplement regimen, always seek the advice of a healthcare professional if you have any concerns or specific medical issues.

CHAPTER NINE

Including Green Tea Extract In Your Everyday Activities

Because green tea extract has so many potential health benefits, incorporating it into your daily routine can be a wise and healthy decision. Because of its antioxidant qualities and capacity to enhance general well-being, this natural supplement has grown in popularity over time. But, to get the most out of green tea extract, you must understand how to use it in your daily routine.

Making The Ideal Cup Of Tea

Making a cup of green tea is still, for many, the most classic and simple approach to include this extract in your daily routine. The method is quite easy to follow: start with high-quality green tea bags or leaves, then steep them for a few minutes in hot water that isn't boiling.

It is important to avoid over-brewing, as this may result in an unpleasant flavor and could reduce the health advantages. Generally speaking, green tea is best served between 170-185°F (77-85°C).

Although making a cup of green tea may seem simple, it's a fun and delightful method to incorporate this extract into your daily routine.

After a hectic day, the routine of making and enjoying a cup of tea can be soothing and help you relax.

This traditional method is a healthy option for people who want a more natural approach to their dietary supplements because it lets you experience the entire range of green tea's flavor and components.

Using Green Tea In Cooking

You may also incorporate green tea extract into your routine by experimenting with food and cookery. You may give meals the distinct flavor and possible health advantages of this extract by adding matcha powder or green tea leaves to your recipes. The earthy, slightly bitter flavor of green tea goes well with a variety of recipes, both savory and sweet.

Green tea leaves, for example, can be used to flavor rice. Matcha powder can also be added to smoothies, baked goods, and even savory recipes like marinades and soups. There are countless ways to include green tea in your cuisine, and doing so can be an enjoyable and inventive way to reap its health benefits and give your dishes a distinctive touch.

Complementary Recipes

Green tea extract can be added to food and beverages as well as supplements, which makes it simple to include into your daily routine in a convenient and well-planned manner. The active ingredients in green tea, such as polyphenols and catechins, are supplied in standardized doses by these supplements, which are usually available as soft gels or capsules.

Choosing a green tea extract supplement requires careful consideration of reliable brands that offer superior products. It's also a good idea to speak with a healthcare provider to figure out the proper dosage and make sure the supplement supports your unique health objectives. Green tea pills are a popular option for people looking for a simpler approach to adding green tea extract to their daily routine because of their possible antioxidant, metabolism-boosting, and general health advantages.

Including green tea extract in your regular regimen can be a good way to support general health and take advantage of its possible benefits. There's no shortage of methods to include this extract into your daily routine, be it through supplement formulations, culinary trials, or the classic brewing approach.

Through experimentation and customization, you may optimize the possible health advantages of the green tea extract and improve your daily regimen.

CHAPTER TEN

The Interaction Of Green Tea Extract With Other Substances

A well-liked nutritional supplement, green tea extract has garnered attention due to its possible health advantages. It is made from Camellia sinensis plant leaves and is rich in bioactive substances, such as catechins, which are polyphenols. These substances are thought to contribute to the possible health benefits of green tea extract because of their antioxidant qualities. But it's crucial to know how green tea extract reacts with other drugs, alcohol, and caffeine, among other things.

Content Of Caffeine

Caffeine is one prominent ingredient in green tea extract. Even while green tea typically contains less caffeine than coffee, it can nevertheless be stimulating. People who are sensitive to caffeine should be mindful of their total caffeine intake when taking green tea extract. Overindulgence in caffeine can have negative consequences like jitters, elevated heart rate, and insomnia. To prevent overstimulation, those who currently use caffeine from other sources, such as coffee or energy drinks, should keep an eye on their daily caffeine intake overall.

Interactions With Medication

Because green tea extract contains bioactive chemicals, it may interact with different drugs. Green tea extract contains polyphenols, particularly catechins, which can obstruct the absorption and metabolism of some medications.

For instance, they might have an impact on iron's bioavailability and lessen the potency of iron supplements. To maximize iron absorption, it is advised to take iron supplements apart from green tea extract.

Additionally, because some of the chemicals in green tea extract can activate or inhibit liver enzymes involved in drug metabolism, it may interact with drugs that are processed by the liver.

This may result in changes to bloodstream drug concentrations, which could have an impact on the effectiveness and safety of prescription drugs. Before incorporating green tea extract into their regimen, people on prescription drugs should speak with their doctor to be sure there are no possible interactions that can reduce the medication's therapeutic benefits.

Drinking alcohol in addition to green tea extract should also be done carefully. Green tea and alcohol both contain bioactive chemicals that, when combined, can enhance each other's effects.

Green tea extract may speed up the body's metabolism of alcohol, which could result in drunkenness more quickly. Individual tolerance levels and the amount of alcohol and green tea extract ingested can all affect how this interaction behaves.

 People who use alcohol should cut back on it and pay attention to how their bodies react to the combination to prevent unpleasant surprises.

The polyphenol concentration of green tea extract makes it a dietary supplement with numerous potential health advantages. It's crucial to understand how it interacts with other drugs, though.

Those who are sensitive to caffeine or who ingest it from other sources may be impacted by the amount of caffeine in green tea extract. Furthermore, green tea extract can affect how well pharmaceuticals work in conjunction with other prescriptions, especially when iron supplements and liver-metabolized drugs are involved.

 Lastly, using alcohol and green tea extract together may have amplified effects, so proceed with caution. Before introducing green tea extract into your daily routine, as with any dietary supplement, it is essential to speak with a healthcare provider, particularly if you are using medication or have specific health issues.

CHAPTER ELEVEN

Myths & Misconceptions Regarding Green Tea Extract

Because of its possible health benefits, green tea extract, which is made from the leaves of the Camellia sinensis plant, has become more and more popular in recent years. Like many nutritional supplements, though, it has also given rise to a lot of myths and false beliefs.

To distinguish fact from fiction, we shall dispel some common misconceptions about green tea extract in this debate and provide light on the available scientific data.

Green Tea Extract Can Help You Lose Weight Without Effort: One of the most widespread myths is that green tea extract works like magic to help people lose weight without requiring them to make dietary or exercise modifications. Although substances found in green tea extract, such as catechins, may have a slight thermogenic effect and encourage fat burning, their contribution to weight loss is quite small. It shouldn't be seen as a magic cure, but rather as an additional tool in a more comprehensive weight-management plan.

Not Every Green Tea Extract Supplement Is Designed Equally? Not every green tea extract supplement is made equally. There is a false belief that all products bearing the label "green tea extract" will have the same advantages. The truth is that there can be big differences in these supplements' composition and quality.

To make sure you are getting what you anticipate, it is crucial to select products from reliable manufacturers and look for standardized extracts with known quantities of active ingredients, especially catechins, on the label.

The idea that green tea extract is completely risk-free and devoid of adverse effects is another common misunderstanding.

While moderate consumption of green tea as part of a tea or diet is usually seen to be healthy, large dosages of the supplement can have negative consequences as well, such as liver damage, digestive issues, and drug interactions. Before beginning any new supplement regimen, it is imperative to speak with a healthcare provider, particularly if you have underlying medical concerns or are currently taking other medications.

Green Tea Extract Can Treat Any Illness Some people think that green tea extract can treat any illness, including diabetes, heart disease, and cancer. It's important to realize that while there is encouraging evidence indicating that the bioactive components in green tea may have health advantages, they should never be used in place of medical care. It is best to think of green tea extract as a component of a comprehensive strategy for preserving and enhancing health.

There is a common misperception that boosting the dosage of green tea extract will result in more advantages. However, as was already indicated, excessive intake may not always offer additional benefits and may even pose health dangers. Depending on personal circumstances, the ideal dosage for green tea extract may differ, therefore it's best to speak with a healthcare professional or adhere to the suggested dosage guidelines on the supplement's label.

Is Green Tea Extract a Miracle Anti-Aging Solution? No, green tea is not a magical anti-aging potion, but its antioxidants and possible anti-inflammatory qualities can benefit skin health and general well-being. The process of aging is complicated and impacted by several environmental and genetic variables. While green tea extract may help maintain the health of the skin, it cannot completely halt or reverse the aging process.

Green tea extract is a potentially beneficial dietary supplement, but it's important to approach it knowing its limitations and the common myths and misconceptions around it. Maintaining a balanced view of green tea extract's function in your overall health and wellness, consulting with healthcare specialists, and depending on scientific research are the keys to making informed judgments about utilizing it.

Our knowledge of the possible uses and health advantages of green tea extract supplementation is expected to grow substantially as a result of upcoming studies and advancements in the field. Because of the increased interest in this natural substance due to its alleged medicinal benefits, scientists are keen to investigate new directions and deepen their understanding to fully realize this product's potential.

The ongoing study of the bioactive substances found in green tea extracts is one interesting direction for future research. Although catechins—in particular, epigallocatechin gallate, or EGCG—have garnered a lot of interest, more research into other substances like polyphenols, theanine, and caffeine could provide insightful information. A more thorough knowledge of how green tea extracts affect human health may be obtained by identifying and comprehending the synergistic effects of these substances.

Furthermore, more investigation into the molecular processes behind the possible health advantages of green tea extract is probably in store. The methods by which these bioactive substances interact with particular biological processes, such as those about oxidative stress, inflammation, and metabolism, will become clearer with the aid of sophisticated molecular and cellular approaches. The creation of more specialized interventions for a range of medical diseases can be guided by this knowledge.

The development of green tea extract supplement formulations and delivery systems will be another area of future research emphasis. Researchers will probably look at new encapsulation techniques to improve these chemicals' release characteristics, stability, and bioavailability. With the least amount of possible negative effects, this invention can guarantee that people get the most out of taking green tea supplements.

Determining the long-term effects of supplementing with green tea extract on human health would require extensive clinical trials and epidemiological research. Researchers can gain a greater understanding of the preventive and therapeutic possibilities of data in chronic diseases such as cancer, diabetes, cardiovascular disease, and neurodegenerative disorders as more data becomes available.

The idea of customized diets and care regimens will be crucial to advancements down the road. Determining the genetic and metabolic components that affect a person's reaction to taking supplements of green tea extract might result in customized advice that optimizes its advantages for particular demographics.

it is essential to investigate any possible negative effects and combinations of green tea extract with other dietary ingredients or prescription drugs. Future studies will concentrate on the safety profile of these supplements, making sure that any associated dangers are well-understood and that advice is supported by data.

Finally, there may be uses for green tea extract supplements outside of just promoting general health. We will look more closely into its possibilities in the areas of mental health, weight control, and sports performance. Thorough clinical trials and a thorough investigation of its mechanisms of action in these particular circumstances will be necessary for this.

Exciting prospects await green tea extract supplementation research in the future. We may anticipate the creation of more potent, secure, and focused uses for this natural product in enhancing human health and well-being as our knowledge of its bioactive components and molecular mechanisms expands and as individualized techniques become more popular.

Recent years have seen a notable increase in the popularity of green tea extract supplements because of the many positive reviews and success stories linked to their use. Numerous people who have included green tea extract in their daily routines have reported a wide range of health benefits and favorable outcomes. The potential benefits of this supplement are highlighted in these testimonials, which makes it a desirable choice for people looking to improve their health and well-being.

Weight control is a popular success story involving green tea extract supplements. Numerous individuals have reported that incorporating these supplements into their diets resulted in a higher metabolism and weight loss. Epigallocatechin gallate (EGCG), the main ingredient in green tea extract, is frequently blamed for this effect since it may enhance calorie expenditure and encourage fat oxidation.

The ability of green tea extract to increase energy and improve mental alertness has also drawn attention. Customers have reported feeling more energized and less fatigued, which is probably because green tea extract contains caffeine. But it's important to take this supplement sparingly because too much caffeine might cause negative effects like jitters and insomnia.

Regarding general well-being, several people have reported that green tea extract lowers their chance of developing chronic illnesses. Green tea's antioxidants, especially EGCG, are well-known for their ability to help the body fight inflammation and oxidative stress. This has led to assertions that people who frequently use green tea extract supplements have better blood sugar control, decreased cancer risk, and enhanced cardiovascular health.

Green tea extract's benefits for the skin are frequently mentioned in testimonials. This supplement's antioxidant qualities may help shield the skin from UV ray damage and other environmental stresses, possibly resulting in a more young and radiant complexion. While these testimonies appear encouraging, it's crucial to remember that every person's experience is unique, and green tea extract supplements shouldn't be used in place of good skincare practices and sun protection.

Conclusion

Numerous endorsements and success stories from people who have included green tea extract supplements into their daily routines attest to the wide range of possible health benefits they offer. Green tea extract is well known for its many benefits, including helping people lose weight, increasing energy, sharpening mental focus, and maybe lowering their chance of developing chronic illnesses.

It's important to read these testimonials critically and keep in mind that different people will react differently to green tea extract. A person may not have the same results from something that works for them. Before incorporating any new supplement into your routine, you must speak with a healthcare provider. They can offer tailored guidance and guarantee that the supplement won't interfere with any existing medical issues or prescriptions.

Although there has been much appreciation for green tea extract supplements' potential health advantages, it is crucial to utilize them in conjunction with a balanced and healthy lifestyle. Green tea extract can be a beneficial supplement to a wellness regimen when taken carefully and under expert advice.